Diabetic Diet For Kids: A Parent's Guide to Supporting your Child's Health with a Diabetic Friendly Diet

Charles Kim

Table of content

Chapter 1

Understanding Diabetes

Diabetes is a chronic medical condition that affects the body's ability to regulate blood sugar levels. The disease is characterized by high levels of glucose in the blood, which can cause a wide range of complications if left untreated. In this article, we will discuss the causes, symptoms, diagnosis, and treatment options for diabetes.

Causes of Diabetes

There are two main types of diabetes: Type 1 and Type 2. Type 1 diabetes is an autoimmune disorder that typically develops in childhood or adolescence. It occurs when the immune system attacks and destroys the insulin-producing cells in the pancreas, which leads to a complete deficiency of insulin. Insulin is a hormone that is necessary for the body to process glucose, so without insulin, glucose cannot enter the body's cells and remains in the bloodstream.

Type 2 diabetes is a metabolic disorder that typically develops in adulthood, although it is becoming increasingly common in younger individuals. In this type of diabetes, the body becomes resistant to insulin, which means that it is unable to use insulin effectively to process glucose. Over time, the pancreas may also become less able to produce enough insulin to keep blood sugar levels in check.

There are several risk factors that can increase the likelihood of developing diabetes, including:

- Being overweight or obese
- Having a family history of diabetes
- Living a sedentary lifestyle
- Eating a diet that is high in processed foods and sugar
- Having high blood pressure or high cholesterol
- Being over the age of 45

- Having a history of gestational diabetes

Symptoms of Diabetes

The symptoms of diabetes can vary depending on the type of diabetes and the severity of the condition. Some common symptoms of diabetes include:

- Increased thirst and hunger
- Frequent urination
- Fatigue and weakness
- Blurred vision
- Slow-healing wounds or infections
- Tingling or numbness in the hands or feet
- Unexplained weight loss

If you experience any of these symptoms, it is important to speak with your healthcare provider to determine the underlying cause and receive appropriate treatment.

Diagnosis of Diabetes

Diabetes is typically diagnosed through blood tests that measure the level of glucose in the blood. If your healthcare provider suspects that you may have diabetes, they may perform one or more of the following tests:

- Fasting blood sugar test: This test measures your blood sugar level after fasting for at least 8 hours.
- A1C test: This test measures your average blood sugar level over the past 2-3 months.

- Oral glucose tolerance test: This test measures your blood sugar level before and after drinking a sugary drink.

If your blood sugar level is consistently elevated, your healthcare provider will likely diagnose you with diabetes and work with you to develop a treatment plan.

Treatment of Diabetes

The goal of diabetes treatment is to manage blood sugar levels and prevent complications. Treatment options will vary depending on the type and severity of diabetes, but may include:

- **Lifestyle changes**: Eating a healthy diet, getting regular exercise, and maintaining a healthy weight can all help to manage blood sugar levels.
- **Medications**: Depending on the type of diabetes, your healthcare provider may prescribe medications to help regulate blood sugar levels. This may include insulin injections or oral medications that help the body use insulin more effectively.
- **Continuous glucose monitoring:** Some individuals with diabetes may benefit from continuous glucose monitoring, which uses a small sensor inserted under the skin to measure blood sugar levels continuously throughout the day.

It is important to work closely with your healthcare provider to develop a personalized treatment plan that meets your individual needs.

Complications of Diabetes

If left untreated, diabetes can lead to a wide range of complications, including:

- Cardiovascular disease
- Kidney damage
- Eye damage and vision loss
- Nerve damage

Diabetes in children

Diabetes in children is diagnosed using the same diagnostic criteria as in adults. However, the symptoms of diabetes in children may be less obvious, making it more challenging to diagnose the condition. In this article, we will discuss the diagnosis of diabetes in children, including the tests used and the criteria for diagnosis.

Symptoms of Diabetes in Children

The symptoms of diabetes in children are similar to those in adults and include:

- Frequent urination
- Excessive thirst
- Unexplained weight loss
- Fatigue
- Blurred vision
- Irritability or mood changes
- Bedwetting (in younger children)

It is important to note that some of these symptoms may also be present in other conditions, so it is essential to seek medical attention if your child is experiencing any of these symptoms.

Diagnostic Criteria for Diabetes in Children

The diagnostic criteria for diabetes in children are the same as for adults, as recommended by the American Diabetes Association. The criteria include:

A fasting blood sugar level of 126 mg/dL or higher

A random blood sugar level of 200 mg/dL or higher, along with symptoms of diabetes

A hemoglobin A1C level of 6.5% or higher

In addition to these diagnostic criteria, your healthcare provider may also perform additional tests to confirm a diagnosis of diabetes, including:

- Urine test: A urine test can detect the presence of glucose in the urine, which is a sign of high blood sugar levels.
- Oral glucose tolerance test: This test involves drinking a sugary drink, and then measuring blood sugar levels over time to see how the body responds to the sugar.

It is important to note that children may experience temporary spikes in blood sugar levels due to illness or stress, which can lead to a false diagnosis of diabetes. For this reason, your healthcare provider may perform additional tests to confirm a diagnosis of diabetes and rule out other potential causes of high blood sugar levels.

Treatment of Diabetes in Children

The treatment of diabetes in children is similar to that in adults, and includes:

- Insulin therapy: Children with type 1 diabetes require insulin injections to regulate their blood sugar levels. Depending on the child's age and ability to self-administer insulin, parents may need to administer insulin injections or use an insulin pump.

- Blood sugar monitoring: Children with diabetes need to monitor their blood sugar levels regularly to adjust their insulin dosage and prevent complications.
- Lifestyle changes: Eating a healthy diet and engaging in regular physical activity can help children with diabetes manage their blood sugar levels and reduce the risk of complications.

It is important to work closely with your healthcare provider to develop a personalized treatment plan that meets your child's individual needs.

In conclusion, the diagnosis of diabetes in children is based on the same criteria as in adults, and includes blood sugar tests and other diagnostic tests. Early diagnosis and treatment are essential to prevent complications and ensure that children with diabetes can lead healthy, active lives. Parents and caregivers should be aware of the symptoms of diabetes in children and seek medical attention if they suspect that their child may have the condition.

Chapter 2

Importance of Diet

Diet plays a crucial role in managing diabetes in children. A healthy diet can help children with diabetes control their blood sugar levels, maintain a healthy weight, and reduce the risk of complications. In this article, we will discuss the importance of diet for children with diabetes, including recommended foods and meal planning strategies.

What should children with diabetes eat?

The key to a healthy diet for children with diabetes is to focus on nutrient-dense foods that provide energy, vitamins, and minerals without causing a sharp rise in blood sugar levels. Some recommended foods for children with diabetes include:

- **Non-starchy vegetables**: Vegetables such as broccoli, carrots, spinach, and cucumbers are low in carbohydrates and high in fiber, making them an excellent choice for children with diabetes.
- **Whole grains:** Whole grains such as brown rice, whole wheat bread, and quinoa are rich in fiber and complex carbohydrates, which help regulate blood sugar levels.
- **Lean proteins:** Lean proteins such as chicken, fish, turkey, and tofu are low in saturated fat and provide essential amino acids needed for growth and development.
- **Low-fat dairy products:** Low-fat dairy products such as milk, cheese, and yogurt are a good source of calcium, which is important for bone health.
- **Fruits:** Fruits such as berries, apples, and citrus fruits are high in fiber and vitamins, but should be eaten in moderation due to their natural sugar content.

How food affect the blood sugar level of diabetic children

For children with diabetes, it is important to monitor and control their blood sugar levels to prevent complications and promote overall health. Food choices can have a significant impact on blood sugar levels, so it is essential to understand how different foods affect glucose levels.

Carbohydrates are the primary nutrient that affects blood sugar levels. When a child consumes carbohydrates, they are broken down into glucose, which enters the bloodstream and raises blood sugar levels. This is why monitoring carbohydrate intake is crucial for diabetic children.

Foods with a high glycemic index (GI) can cause a rapid increase in blood sugar levels. High GI foods include white bread, white rice, sugary drinks, candy, and other foods with added sugars. These foods should be limited in a diabetic child's diet, as they can cause blood sugar spikes and increase the risk of long-term complications.On the other hand, foods with a low glycemic index (GI) are absorbed more slowly and can help stabilize blood sugar levels. Low GI foods include

fruits, vegetables, whole grains, and legumes. These foods are an excellent source of nutrients, fiber, and carbohydrates, making them a healthy choice for diabetic children.In addition to monitoring carbohydrate intake and choosing low GI foods, diabetic children should also consider portion sizes and meal timing. Eating smaller, more frequent meals throughout the day can help prevent blood sugar spikes and promote more stable glucose levels. It is also essential to balance carbohydrate intake with protein and healthy fats to slow the absorption of carbohydrates and promote satiety.

Finally, it is important to work with a healthcare professional or registered dietitian to develop a personalized meal plan for a diabetic child. They can help guide food choices, recommend portion sizes, and monitor blood sugar levels to ensure that the child is maintaining healthy glucose levels.

In summary, food choices can have a significant impact on blood sugar levels in diabetic children. By monitoring carbohydrate intake, choosing low GI foods, and balancing meals with protein and healthy fats, it is possible to promote stable glucose levels and prevent complications. Working with a healthcare professional or registered dietitian is crucial to developing a personalized meal plan that meets the child's unique needs.

Importance of Balancing carbohydrates, proteins, and fats in meals for diabetic children

Balancing carbohydrates, proteins, and fats in meals is crucial for diabetic children as it can help them manage their blood sugar levels, prevent complications, and maintain a healthy weight. Diabetes is a condition where the body cannot properly use and store glucose, which is the primary source of energy for the body. This results in high blood sugar levels, which can cause a range of health problems if left uncontrolled.

Here are some reasons why balancing carbs, proteins, and fats is essential for diabetic children:

- Regulating blood sugar levels: Carbohydrates are broken down into glucose, which is then used as energy by the body. However, in diabetic children, this process can become disrupted, leading to high blood sugar levels. By balancing carbohydrates with proteins and fats, the absorption of glucose can be slowed down, preventing spikes in blood sugar levels.
- Preventing complications: High blood sugar levels can cause a range of health problems, including nerve damage, kidney damage, and heart disease. By balancing carbs, proteins, and fats, diabetic children can reduce the risk of developing these complications and lead a healthier life.

- Managing weight: Children with diabetes are more likely to be overweight or obese, which can worsen their condition. Balancing carbohydrates with proteins and fats can help diabetic children maintain a healthy weight, as protein and fat are more filling and can help control appetite.
- Ensuring proper nutrition: A balanced meal that includes carbs, proteins, and fats can provide the body with all the necessary nutrients it needs to function properly. Diabetic children may be at risk of nutrient deficiencies due to restricted food choices or poor appetite, so it's important to make every meal count.
- So how can parents ensure that their diabetic children are getting a balanced diet? Here are some tips:
- Choose carbohydrates wisely: Instead of sugary or processed carbs, opt for whole-grain bread, rice, and pasta, as well as fruits, vegetables, and legumes. These foods contain fiber, which slows down the absorption of glucose and helps regulate blood sugar levels.
- Include protein at every meal: Protein can help balance blood sugar levels and control appetite. Good sources of protein include lean meats, poultry, fish, eggs, dairy products, nuts, and seeds.
- Incorporate healthy fats: Healthy fats, such as those found in nuts, seeds, avocado, and olive oil, can help lower inflammation and improve insulin sensitivity. However, it's important to limit saturated and trans fats, which can raise cholesterol levels and increase the risk of heart disease.
- Work with a dietitian: A registered dietitian can help parents develop a balanced meal plan for their diabetic child, taking into account their age, weight, activity level, and food

preferences. They can also provide guidance on portion sizes, meal timing, and snacking.

In conclusion, balancing carbohydrates, proteins, and fats in meals is essential for diabetic children to manage their blood sugar levels, prevent complications, and maintain a healthy weight. With the right guidance and support, parents can help their children thrive despite their diabetes diagnosis.

Chapter 3

Meal planning

Meal planning is a critical aspect of managing diabetes in children. A healthy and balanced diet can help regulate blood sugar levels, reduce the risk of complications, and ensure that your child gets the essential nutrients they need to grow and thrive. In this section, we'll discuss some key strategies for meal planning for diabetic children.

- **Focus on Carbohydrates**: Carbohydrates are the main source of energy for the body, but they also have a significant impact on blood sugar levels. It's essential to choose healthy carbohydrates that are high in fiber and low in simple sugars. Good carbohydrate sources include whole grains, vegetables, fruits, legumes, and low-fat dairy products. You should also aim to balance the amount of carbohydrates with the amount of protein and fat in each meal.

- **Plan Meals in Advance**: Planning meals in advance can help you ensure that your child's diet is well-balanced and meets their nutritional needs. It can also help you avoid the temptation to make unhealthy food choices when you're short on time or don't feel like cooking. Try to plan your meals for the week ahead, taking into account your child's schedule, preferences, and any special occasions.

- **Portion Control:** Portion control is important for maintaining a healthy weight and regulating blood sugar levels. A good rule of thumb is to fill half of your child's plate with non-starchy vegetables, a quarter with lean protein, and a quarter with healthy carbohydrates. You can use measuring cups, food scales, or visual aids (like a deck of cards) to help you estimate portion sizes.

- **Snacks:** Healthy snacks can help keep your child's blood sugar levels stable throughout the day. Choose snacks that are high in fiber and protein, such as fresh fruit, raw vegetables, nuts, and low-fat cheese. You can also try making your own diabetic-friendly snacks, like homemade trail mix or low-carb muffins.
- **Avoid Processed Foods**: Processed foods are often high in sodium,, and unhealthy fats, which can lead to weight gain and blood sugar spikes. Instead, focus on whole, nutrient-dense foods that are low in added sugars and unhealthy fats. Choose fresh or frozen fruits and vegetables, lean proteins, and healthy fats like nuts, seeds, and avocados.
- **Get Creative with Recipes:** A healthy diabetic diet doesn't have to be bland or boring. Get creative with your recipes by using spices, herbs, and healthy sauces to add flavor to your meals. Experiment with new recipes and ingredients to keep things interesting and avoid falling into a rut.
- **Seek Professional Advice:** If you're struggling with meal planning or need more guidance, consider seeking advice from a registered dietitian who specializes in diabetes. A dietitian can help you develop a personalized meal plan that meets your child's individual needs and preferences.

why it's important to balance carbs, proteins and fats in meals for diabetic children.

Balancing carbohydrates, proteins, and fats in meals is crucial for diabetic children as it can help them manage their blood sugar levels, prevent complications, and maintain a healthy weight. Diabetes is a condition where the body cannot properly use and store glucose, which is the primary source of energy for the body. This results in high blood sugar levels, which can cause a range of health problems if left uncontrolled.Here are some reasons why balancing carbs, proteins, and fats is essential for diabetic children:

- **Regulating blood sugar levels**: Carbohydrates are broken down into glucose, which is then used as energy by the body. However, in diabetic children, this process can become disrupted, leading to high blood sugar levels. By balancing carbohydrates with proteins and fats, the absorption of glucose can be slowed down, preventing spikes in blood sugar levels.
- **Preventing complications:** High blood sugar levels can cause a range of health problems, including nerve damage, kidney damage, and heart disease. By balancing carbs, proteins, and fats, diabetic children can reduce the risk of developing these complications and lead a healthier life.
- **Managing weight:** Children with diabetes are more likely to be overweight or obese, which can worsen their condition. Balancing carbohydrates with proteins and fats can help diabetic children maintain a healthy weight, as protein and fat are more filling and can help control appetite.
- **Ensuring proper nutrition:** A balanced meal that includes carbs, proteins, and fats can provide the body with all the necessary nutrients it needs to function properly. Diabetic children may be at risk of nutrient deficiencies due to restricted food choices or poor appetite, so it's important to make every meal count.

So how can parents ensure that their diabetic children are getting a balanced diet? Here are some tips:

- **Choose carbohydrates wisely**: Instead of sugary or processed carbs, opt for whole-grain bread, rice, and pasta, as well as fruits, vegetables, and legumes. These foods contain fiber, which slows down the absorption of glucose and helps regulate blood sugar levels.
- **Include protein at every meal**: Protein can help balance blood sugar levels and control appetite. Good sources of protein include lean meats, poultry, fish, eggs, dairy products, nuts, and seeds.
- **Incorporate healthy fats**: Healthy fats, such as those found in nuts, seeds, avocado, and olive oil, can help lower inflammation and improve insulin sensitivity. However, it's important to limit saturated and trans fats, which can raise cholesterol levels and increase the risk of heart disease.
- **Work with a dietitian:** A registered dietitian can help parents develop a balanced meal plan for their diabetic child, taking into account their age, weight, activity level, and food preferences. They can also provide guidance on portion sizes, meal timing, and snacking.

In conclusion, balancing carbohydrates, proteins, and fats in meals is essential for diabetic children to manage their blood sugar levels, prevent complications, and maintain a healthy weight. With the right guidance and support, parents can help their children thrive despite their diabetes diagnosis.

List of food that are good for managing good blood sugar levels for kids with diabetes

Managing blood sugar levels in children with diabetes can be challenging, especially when it comes to their diet. It is important to provide them with a balanced diet that is low in sugar and high in fiber and complex carbohydrates. Here are some foods that are good for managing blood sugar levels in kids with diabetes:

- **Non-Starchy Vegetables:** Non-starchy vegetables such as broccoli, cauliflower, bell peppers, spinach, and kale are low in calories and carbohydrates, high in fiber, and rich in important vitamins and minerals. They have a low glycemic index, meaning they do not cause a significant increase in blood sugar levels.
- **Whole Grains:** Whole grains like brown rice, quinoa, and whole wheat bread are high in fiber and complex carbohydrates, which can help regulate blood sugar levels. They also provide important vitamins and minerals.
- **Legumes**: Legumes such as beans, lentils, and chickpeas are a good source of protein, fiber, and complex carbohydrates. They have a low glycemic index and can help with weight management, which is important for managing blood sugar levels.
- **Fruits**: Fruits such as apples, berries, and citrus fruits are a good source of fiber, vitamins, and minerals. They also contain natural sugars, so it is important to limit the amount consumed. Eating whole fruits instead of drinking fruit juice can help with blood sugar management.
- **Nuts and Seeds:** Nuts and seeds like almonds, walnuts, chia seeds, and flaxseeds are a good source of healthy fats, protein, and fiber. They can help slow down the absorption of

carbohydrates, which can help with blood sugar management. However, it is important to keep portion sizes in mind as they are high in calories.

- **Lean Proteins:** Lean proteins such as chicken, turkey, fish, and tofu are a good source of protein without the added saturated fat found in red meats. Protein can help regulate blood sugar levels and help with weight management.
- **Low-Fat Dairy**: Low-fat dairy products like milk, yogurt, and cheese are a good source of calcium and protein. They also have a low glycemic index, meaning they do not cause a significant increase in blood sugar levels.

It is important to monitor the portion sizes of all foods, including those that are considered healthy. Eating large portions of even healthy foods can cause a spike in blood sugar levels. It is also important to talk to a healthcare provider or a registered dietitian to create a personalized meal plan based on the child's individual needs and preferences.Children with diabetes may also benefit from eating smaller, more frequent meals throughout the day instead of larger meals. This can help regulate blood sugar levels and prevent spikes and drops. Snacks that are high in protein and fiber, such as hummus and carrots or apple slices with almond butter, can also help manage blood sugar levels between meals.

It is important for children with diabetes to have a healthy relationship with food and to not feel restricted or deprived. Working with a healthcare provider and a registered dietitian can help ensure that children with diabetes are getting the nutrients they need while managing their blood sugar levels.

Chapter 4

Snacks And Desserts

Diabetes is a chronic medical condition characterized by high levels of blood sugar, which can cause a range of complications if left untreated. For children with diabetes, it's important to maintain stable blood sugar levels through a balanced and nutritious diet. While it may seem challenging to find healthy snacks and desserts that are suitable for diabetic children, there are plenty of delicious and wholesome options available. In this article, we'll explore some healthy snack and dessert ideas for diabetic children.

Healthy Snacks for Diabetic Children:

- **Fresh Fruits:** Fresh fruits like apples, pears, berries, and citrus fruits are a great source of vitamins, fiber, and antioxidants, and are low in calories and carbohydrates. These make for a perfect snack for diabetic children as they help to stabilize blood sugar levels.
- **Nuts:** Nuts are a great source of protein, healthy fats, and fiber. They are also low in carbohydrates and can help to lower blood sugar levels. Diabetic children can snack on a handful of almonds, walnuts, or cashews to satisfy hunger cravings.
- **Yogurt:** Yogurt is a great source of protein and probiotics, and can be a healthy snack option for diabetic children. Plain Greek yogurt with no added sugar is an excellent choice as it is low in carbohydrates and provides the necessary protein that helps to stabilize blood sugar levels.
- **Vegetables with Hummus:** Raw vegetables like carrot sticks, cucumber, and bell pepper are a healthy snack option for diabetic children. Pairing them with hummus, a protein-rich dip

made from chickpeas, adds to the nutritional value of the snack and keeps the blood sugar levels stable.

- **Hard-Boiled Eggs:** Hard-boiled eggs are a great source of protein and healthy fats. They are also low in carbohydrates, making them an excellent snack option for diabetic children.

Healthy Desserts for Diabetic Children:

- **Fresh Fruit Salad:** Fresh fruit salad made with a variety of seasonal fruits is a great dessert option for diabetic children. It is low in calories and carbohydrates and provides essential vitamins, minerals, and fiber.
- **Homemade Popsicles:** Homemade popsicles made with natural sweeteners like stevia, honey, or fruit juice are a great alternative to store-bought popsicles that are often high in sugar. You can make popsicles with fruits like berries, kiwi, or mango to provide a sweet and refreshing treat for diabetic children.
- **Chia Seed Pudding:** Chia seed pudding made with unsweetened almond milk, chia seeds, and fresh fruit is a healthy dessert option for diabetic children. Chia seeds are rich in fiber, healthy fats, and protein, and can help to stabilize blood sugar levels.
- **Frozen Yogurt:** Frozen yogurt made with plain Greek yogurt, fresh fruit, and natural sweeteners like stevia or honey is a healthier alternative to ice cream. It provides the necessary protein, vitamins, and minerals and is low in calories and carbohydrates.

- **Dark Chocolate:** Dark chocolate with a high cocoa content is a healthy dessert option for diabetic children. It is low in sugar and provides essential antioxidants that can help to improve heart health.

Recipes For Diabetic-Friendly Desserts That Kids Will Love.

Diabetes is a chronic condition that requires careful management, particularly when it comes to diet. Children with diabetes can still enjoy desserts, but it's important to choose recipes that are low in sugar and carbohydrates. Here are some delicious and diabetic-friendly dessert recipes that kids will love.

Sugar-Free Apple Crumble

Ingredients:

6 apples, peeled and chopped

1 tsp cinnamon

1/2 tsp nutmeg

1/2 cup almond flour

1/2 cup rolled oats

1/2 cup chopped pecans

1/4 cup melted butter

1/4 cup granulated stevia

Instructions:

Preheat the oven to 350°F.

In a mixing bowl, mix together the apples, cinnamon, and nutmeg.

In a separate bowl, mix together the almond flour, rolled oats, pecans, melted butter, and granulated stevia.

Pour the apple mixture into a baking dish, and top with the almond flour mixture.

Bake for 35-40 minutes, or until the crumble is golden brown and the apples are soft.

Chocolate Avocado Pudding

Ingredients:

2 ripe avocados

1/2 cup unsweetened cocoa powder

1/2 cup unsweetened almond milk

1/4 cup granulated stevia

1 tsp vanilla extract

Instructions:

In a food processor or blender, blend together the avocados, cocoa powder, almond milk, granulated stevia, and vanilla extract until smooth.

Divide the pudding into serving cups or bowls and chill in the refrigerator for at least 1 hour before serving.

Low-Carb Peanut Butter Cookies

Ingredients:

1 cup natural peanut butter

1/2 cup granulated stevia

1 egg

1 tsp vanilla extract

1/2 tsp baking soda

Instructions:

Preheat the oven to 350°F.

In a mixing bowl, whisk together the peanut butter, granulated stevia, egg, vanilla extract, and baking soda until well combined.

Roll the dough into balls and place them onto a baking sheet lined with parchment paper.

Use a fork to flatten the balls into cookies.

Bake for 10-12 minutes or until the edges of the cookies are lightly browned.

Cool the cookies on the baking sheet for 5 minutes, then transfer to a wire rack to cool completely.

Raspberry Chia Seed Pudding

Ingredients:

1 cup unsweetened almond milk

1/2 cup fresh raspberries

1/4 cup chia seeds

1/4 cup granulated stevia

1 tsp vanilla extract

Instructions:

In a blender, blend together the almond milk and raspberries until smooth.

Pour the mixture into a mixing bowl and whisk in the chia seeds, granulated stevia, and vanilla extract.

Cover the bowl with plastic wrap and refrigerate for at least 4 hours or overnight.

Serve the pudding chilled, topped with additional raspberries if desired.

Chapter 5

Eating Out

Eating out at restaurants or attending social events can be challenging for children with diabetes as it can be difficult to control the amount and type of food they consume. However, it's still possible to enjoy these occasions while sticking to a diabetic-friendly diet. Here are some tips to help:

- **Plan ahead:** If you know you're going out to eat or attending a social event, plan ahead and check the restaurant menu or ask the host about the food options available. This can help you make informed decisions about what to order or bring your own diabetic-friendly dish to the event.
- **Choose wisely**: When selecting food items, choose options that are low in carbohydrates, sugar, and saturated fats. For example, choose grilled meats or fish instead of fried, and opt for salads or vegetables instead of starchy sides like fries or pasta.
- **Watch portion sizes**: Restaurants often serve large portions, which can make it difficult to control the amount of food consumed. Consider sharing a meal or asking for a takeout container to save some for later.
- **Ask for modifications:** Don't be afraid to ask for modifications to menu items, such as asking for dressing on the side, or requesting grilled instead of breaded chicken. Most restaurants are willing to accommodate special dietary needs.

- **Limit alcohol consumption:** Alcoholic beverages can have a significant impact on blood sugar levels, so it's important to limit consumption or choose low-carb options like light beer or wine.
- **Pack snacks**: If you're going to be out for an extended period of time, pack diabetic-friendly snacks like nuts, fruit, or cheese to prevent low blood sugar episodes.
- **Check blood sugar levels:** It's important to check blood sugar levels regularly while eating out or attending social events to ensure that they are within target ranges. This can help you make adjustments to your food choices and insulin dosages as needed.

Remember, it's possible to enjoy eating out and attending social events while sticking to a diabetic-friendly diet. With some planning and smart choices, children with diabetes can participate in these activities while maintaining good health.

Guidance on how to make health choices for your diabetic kid when dining out

As a parent, making health choices for your diabetic child when dining out can be a daunting task. However, with the right guidance and preparation, you can make informed decisions to ensure that your child maintains a healthy diet while still enjoying the dining experience. Here are some tips to help you make health choices when dining out with your diabetic child:

- **Plan ahead**: Before going out to eat, research the restaurant's menu online to see what options are available. Most restaurants have their menus available online, and some even include nutritional information. This can help you plan ahead and make informed decisions about what to order.

- **Be mindful of portion sizes:** Portion sizes at restaurants are often larger than what is recommended for a diabetic diet. Consider sharing an entrée with your child or ordering a smaller portion size.
- **Choose healthy options:** Look for menu items that are lower in carbohydrates, saturated fat, and added sugars. Choose grilled or baked proteins, such as chicken or fish, and opt for vegetables and salads as sides.
- **Ask for modifications:** Don't be afraid to ask the server if modifications can be made to a dish to make it more suitable for a diabetic diet. For example, ask for sauces and dressings to be served on the side, or for a dish to be prepared without added sugars.
- **Avoid sugary drinks:** Soft drinks and other sugary beverages should be avoided, as they can cause blood sugar levels to spike. Opt for water, unsweetened tea, or diet soda instead.
- **Consider timing:** If your child takes insulin, consider the timing of the meal and the dose of insulin. It is important to discuss this with your child's healthcare provider to ensure that insulin dosages are adjusted accordingly.
- **Pack snacks:** It's always a good idea to have healthy snacks on hand in case of an emergency. Pack some nuts, fruit, or vegetables to bring with you to the restaurant.
- **Communicate with your child:** Talk to your child about healthy eating habits and the importance of making good choices. Encourage them to make their own choices when dining out and to be mindful of portion sizes and sugary foods.

In conclusion, making health choices when dining out with a diabetic child requires planning, preparation, and communication.

Chapter 6

Dealing with challenges

Managing diabetes in children can be challenging for parents, especially when it comes to dealing with peer pressure, managing stress, and sick days. However, with the right guidance and preparation, parents can effectively navigate these challenges and ensure that their diabetic child is healthy and happy. Here are some tips to help parents deal with these challenges:

Dealing with peer pressure

Peer pressure can be a significant challenge for children with diabetes. They may feel excluded from social activities or feel pressured to eat sugary foods. Here are some tips for parents to help their child navigate peer pressure:

- **Educate your child about diabetes:** Teach your child about diabetes and how it affects their body. This will help them understand the importance of making healthy choices and how to communicate their needs to others.
- **Encourage your child to talk to their friends:** Encourage your child to talk to their friends about their diabetes and how it affects their life. This will help their friends understand their needs and support them in making healthy choices.
- **Be supportive:** Offer your child emotional support and encouragement. Let them know that you are proud of them for making healthy choices and that you are there to support them.

Managing stress

Stress can cause blood sugar levels to fluctuate, making it challenging to manage diabetes. Here are some tips for parents to help their child manage stress:

- Encourage physical activity: Regular exercise can help reduce stress and improve blood sugar control. Encourage your child to participate in physical activities they enjoy, such as sports or dancing.
- Teach relaxation techniques: Teach your child relaxation techniques such as deep breathing, meditation, or yoga. These techniques can help reduce stress and promote relaxation.
- Encourage healthy habits: Encourage your child to maintain a healthy lifestyle by eating a balanced diet, getting enough sleep, and managing their time effectively.

Dealing with sick days

Sick days can be especially challenging for children with diabetes. Illness can cause blood sugar levels to fluctuate, and it can be challenging to manage diabetes when your child is not feeling well. Here are some tips for parents to help their child deal with sick days:

- Monitor blood sugar levels frequently: During illness, it's important to monitor blood sugar levels more frequently than usual. This will help you adjust your child's insulin dosage and keep their blood sugar levels in a healthy range.
- Follow sick day rules: Your child's healthcare provider may have specific guidelines for managing diabetes during illness. Follow these guidelines carefully to ensure that your child stays healthy.
- Stay hydrated: Encourage your child to drink plenty of fluids, especially if they have a fever or are vomiting.

Chapter 7

Recipes

It can be challenging to find recipes that are both delicious and healthy for kids with diabetes. However, with a little bit of creativity and planning, it's possible to make meals and snacks that not only taste great but are also nutritious and diabetes-friendly. Here are some easy-to-make recipes that are specifically designed for kids with diabetes.

Banana Oatmeal Pancakes

These pancakes are a great breakfast option for kids with diabetes because they are made with whole-grain oats and bananas, which provide slow-digesting carbs that won't spike blood sugar levels.

Ingredients:

1 cup rolled oats

1 ripe banana, mashed

2 eggs

1 tsp vanilla extract

1 tsp baking powder

1/4 tsp salt

1/4 cup milk (or dairy-free alternative)

Non-stick cooking spray

Instructions:

In a blender or food processor, pulse oats until finely ground.

In a large bowl, mix together mashed banana, eggs, vanilla extract, baking powder, salt, and milk.

Add ground oats to the bowl and stir until well combined.

Heat a non-stick skillet over medium heat and spray with cooking spray.

Spoon batter onto the skillet to make pancakes of desired size.

Cook until bubbles form on the surface of the pancakes, then flip and cook until golden brown on both sides.

Veggie Quesadillas

These veggie quesadillas are packed with flavor and nutrients, making them a great lunch or dinner option for kids with diabetes.

Ingredients:

2 whole-grain tortillas

1/2 cup shredded cheddar cheese

1/2 cup chopped veggies (such as bell peppers, onions, mushrooms, and spinach)

1 tbsp olive oil

Instructions:

Heat a skillet over medium heat and add olive oil.

Add chopped veggies and sauté until tender.

Remove veggies from skillet and set aside.

Place one tortilla in the skillet and sprinkle with half of the shredded cheese.

Add sautéed veggies on top of the cheese.

Sprinkle remaining cheese on top of the veggies.

Place the second tortilla on top of the cheese and veggies.

Cook until the cheese is melted and the tortillas are golden brown on both sides.

Slice into wedges and serve.

Fruit Salad

This fruit salad is a refreshing and healthy snack that kids with diabetes will love.

Ingredients:

1 cup chopped fresh fruit (such as strawberries, blueberries, raspberries, kiwi, and pineapple)

1 tbsp honey

1 tsp fresh lime juice

1/4 tsp ground cinnamon

Instructions:

In a large bowl, mix together chopped fruit.

In a separate bowl, whisk together honey, lime juice, and cinnamon.

Pour honey mixture over the fruit and toss until well combined.

Serve chilled.

In conclusion, these recipes are not only delicious but also designed to help maintain healthy blood sugar levels in kids with diabetes. As with any diet plan for diabetes management, it is essential to consult with a healthcare professional to ensure the proper management of blood sugar levels

Chapter 8

Expert advice

Diabetes is a chronic condition that affects millions of people worldwide, and it can be particularly challenging to manage in children. Fortunately, there are many experts in the field who can offer advice on how to manage diabetes in children effectively. Here are some tips from nutritionists, dietitians, and pediatric endocrinologists:

- **Consistency is key**: Consistency in meal timing, portion sizes, and carbohydrate intake can help regulate blood sugar levels in children with diabetes. It's important to work with a registered dietitian or nutritionist to develop a meal plan that meets the child's nutritional needs and helps keep blood sugar levels stable.
- **Monitor carbohydrate intake**: Carbohydrates are the primary source of glucose in the body, so it's crucial to monitor how much the child is consuming. This can be done by counting carbs or using the glycemic index to choose foods that have a lower impact on blood sugar levels.
- **Encourage physical activity**: Regular exercise can help regulate blood sugar levels, improve insulin sensitivity, and promote overall health in children with diabetes. Encourage children to engage in physical activities they enjoy, such as sports, dancing, or bike riding.
- **Monitor blood sugar levels:** Regular monitoring of blood sugar levels is crucial in managing diabetes in children. Parents should work with their child's healthcare provider to determine the appropriate testing schedule based on the child's age, medication regimen, and overall health.

- **Educate the child and family**: It's important to educate the child and their family about diabetes management, including the importance of monitoring blood sugar levels, taking medications, following a healthy diet, and engaging in physical activity. This education can help the child and their family feel more confident in managing their diabetes and reduce the risk of complications.
- **Seek support**: Living with diabetes can be challenging for both the child and their family, and it's important to seek support from healthcare providers, support groups, and other resources. These resources can offer emotional support, education, and practical tips for managing diabetes in children.

In conclusion, managing diabetes in children requires a multifaceted approach that includes monitoring blood sugar levels, following a healthy diet, engaging in physical activity, and seeking support from healthcare providers and other resources. By working together, children with diabetes and their families can successfully manage this chronic condition and lead healthy, active lives.

Chapter 9

Resources

Here are some resources that parents of children with diabetes may find helpful:

Websites:

American Diabetes Association - Provides information on diabetes management, advocacy, and research.

JDRF (formerly Juvenile Diabetes Research Foundation) - Offers resources for families affected by type 1 diabetes, including advocacy, research, and support.

Beyond Type 1 - A global diabetes community providing information, resources, and support for those affected by type 1 and type 2 diabetes.

Support Groups:

Children with Diabetes - Offers an online community for families affected by type 1 diabetes, including forums, articles, and resources.

Diabetes Sisters - A nonprofit organization offering support groups and resources for women with diabetes, including those with children with diabetes.

T1D Exchange - A patient-centered organization that connects individuals with type 1 diabetes to researchers, healthcare providers, and other resources.

Grocery

Here are some common terms related to diabetes that you may come across:

- Diabetes - A chronic condition in which the body is unable to properly process and use glucose (sugar), resulting in high blood sugar levels.
- Type 1 diabetes - A form of diabetes in which the body's immune system attacks and destroys the cells in the pancreas that produce insulin, resulting in a lack of insulin in the body.
- Type 2 diabetes - A form of diabetes in which the body becomes resistant to insulin or doesn't produce enough insulin to maintain normal blood sugar levels.
- Insulin - A hormone produced by the pancreas that helps regulate blood sugar levels by allowing glucose to enter cells and be used for energy.
- Glucose - A type of sugar that is the primary source of energy for the body's cells.
- Hypoglycemia - A condition in which blood sugar levels are too low, often caused by too much insulin, too little food, or increased physical activity.
- Hyperglycemia - A condition in which blood sugar levels are too high, often caused by a lack of insulin, too much food, or illness.
- HbA1c - A blood test that measures the average blood sugar level over the past 2-3 months, used to monitor long-term diabetes management.

• Carbohydrates - A type of nutrient found in foods such as bread, pasta, and fruit that is broken down into glucose in the body and affects blood sugar levels.

• Ketones - Substances produced by the liver when the body breaks down fat for energy, which can build up in the blood and urine in people with uncontrolled diabetes.

• Diabetic ketoacidosis - A serious complication of diabetes characterized by high blood sugar levels, ketones in the blood and urine, and acidosis.

• Continuous glucose monitoring (CGM) - A device that tracks blood sugar levels continuously and provides real-time information about changes in blood sugar levels.

• Insulin pump - A small, portable device that delivers insulin continuously to the body through a small tube inserted under the skin.

• Diabetic retinopathy - A complication of diabetes that affects the eyes and can cause vision loss.

• Neuropathy - A complication of diabetes that affects the nerves and can cause tingling, numbness, or pain in the hands and feet.